Y0-BDH-814

# KNOWING ABOUT DIABETES

## For Non-Insulin-Dependent Diabetics

*Dr. P. H. Wise MB PhD, FRCP FRACP*

*Consultant Physician*
*Diabetic and Endocrine Clinic*
*Charing Cross Hospital, London*

Second Edition

## foulsham
LONDON • NEW YORK • TORONTO • SYDNEY

# foulsham
Yeovil Road, Slough, Berkshire, SL1 4JH

ISBN 0–572–02021–X

Copyright © 1983 & 1994 P. H. Wise

All rights reserved

The Copyright Act (1956) prohibits (subject to
certain very limited exceptions) the making of
copies of any copyright work or of a substantial
part of such a work, including the making of
copies by photocopying or similar process.
Written permission to make a copy or copies
must therefore normally be obtained from the
publisher in advance. It is advisable also to consult
the publisher if in any doubt as to the legality of
any copying which is to be undertaken.

In this book, the author and editor have done their best to outline the
indicated general treatment for Diabetes (non-Insulin Dependent).
Recommendations are made regarding certain drugs, medications and
preparations.

Different people react to the same treatment, medication, or
preparation in different ways. This book does not purport to answer all
questions about all situations that you or your child may encounter. It
does not attempt to replace your physician.

Neither the editors nor the publishers of this book take responsibility
for any possible consequences from any treatment, action or application
of any medication or preparation to any person reading or following the
information or advice contained in this book. The publication of this
book does not constitute the practice of medicine. The author and
publisher advise that you consult your physician before administering
any medication or undertaking any course of treatment.

Printed in Great Britain by
St Edmundsbury Press Ltd, Bury St Edmunds, Suffolk

# INTRODUCTION: You may have had diabetes for some time: perhaps you already know much of what is in this book. On the other hand, the diagnosis may have just been made, and all that is involved may seem a little bewildering.

This book was written to give you some idea of what diabetes is all about. It tries to answer the type of questions you will ask, both now and in the future. It cannot cover the whole subject, and at the end you will find a list of books for further reading.

There is one thing upon which most authorities agree: the more that diabetics know, the better controlled and the healthier they are likely to be. Never hesitate to ask for further information and help.

# ACKNOWLEDGEMENTS: The author acknowledges with appreciation the constructive criticism of the many patients, nurses and other health professionals who helped to produce this book. Special thanks go to Eleanor McGill for the provision of nutritional information for this book.

# 1 WHAT IS DIABETES?

Diabetes is the name given to a disturbed chemical balance in the body, which can affect a number of different organs. The word diabetes comes from a Greek expression meaning "siphon". It refers to the increased urination and thirst which often occurs in newly diagnosed or uncontrolled cases. These symptoms are due to the high sugar (glucose) content in the urine. The sugar in the urine drags water out with it, the body gets dry and you feel thirsty. All this follows an excessive build-up of glucose in the blood, because there is not enough insulin in your body to deal with it.

Diabetes is due to partial or complete lack of insulin. This hormone is normally released directly into the blood circulation from small pockets of cells

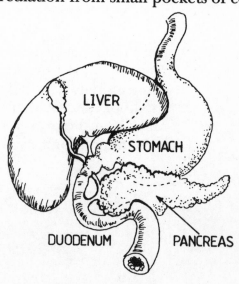

called Islets of Langerhans, which are scattered throughout the pancreas gland (sweetbread). The pancreas rests in the upper abdomen, just beneath the liver, partly behind the stomach in the loop of the duodenum.

The pancreas also produces enzymes, which pass through a duct into the duodenum, where they assist with the digestion of food. This part of the pancreas is only rarely affected in diabetes.

Insulin in usable form was first extracted from animal pancreas in 1921 by two Canadians, Banting and Best. Shortly afterwards it proved successful in the treatment of human diabetes.

About one person in every fifty is diabetic, although only one in four diabetics actually needs insulin for treatment.

## 2 / HOW IS FOOD NORMALLY PROCESSED?

All foods contain one or more of the following energy-producing substances:

carbohydrates
proteins
fats

Once absorbed through the small intestine, they are all processed in the liver, where all three can be converted to glucose, and then released into the bloodstream.

However, carbohydrates, especially in a refined form such as sugar and sweets, are the most rapidly absorbed. Accordingly, they produce the biggest rises in blood glucose level.

Any rises in blood glucose "triggers" the islets of the pancreas to produce insulin, which is then released into the blood vessels passing through the pancreas. In this way, insulin can find its way through the blood circulation to all body tissues.

Although insulin has many different effects, it has one main action: to help glucose in the blood to enter the tissue cells, where it is used as a source of energy. If not required for immediate energy production, insulin also ensures that glucose is converted either to glycogen (for short term energy storage), or to fat (for more long term energy storage).

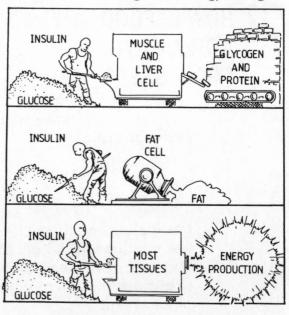

Different tissues use glucose for different purposes.

# 3 WHY DOES DIABETES DEVELOP?

Diabetes is partly inherited, even though you may not be aware that your ancestors were affected. Where diabetes begins before the age of 40, lack of insulin is often complete, perhaps resulting from additional severe damage to the pancreas gland by a virus. Symptoms are then commonly sudden and severe, and in these patients only insulin itself can be used for treatment.

However, in your case (maturity onset, non-insulin dependent, or Type 2 diabetes), insulin deficiency is only mild. In fact, it may only have shown up because you were overweight, or as an effect of ageing or certain drugs. It may also have resulted from a form of stress such as anxiety, infection, or some other illness.

In all of these situations, the body's need for insulin is increased, but cannot be satisfied by the faulty islets. If there is even a mild shortage of insulin, glucose in the blood cannot properly enter tissue cells. Therefore its level in the blood remains above normal even when you have not had anything to eat. After food, blood glucose levels rise higher and remain raised for longer. Such rises of blood sugar above normal are referred to as **hyperglycaemia**.

# HOW DOES UNCONTROLLED DIABETES (HYPERGLYCAEMIA) PRODUCE SYMPTOMS?

a) In the early stages, or if the build-up of glucose is only slight, there **may be no symptoms at all**. As the glucose level rises higher, one or more of the following may occur:

b) The lens of the eye may alter its shape, producing **blurring of vision**

c) High glucose levels in the blood prevent the body's defence against **infection**, particularly in the skin, urine, and lungs. In fact, it may have been a severe or chronic infection which first alerted your doctor that you might have diabetes.

d) By overflowing into the urine (where it can be easily tested) glucose may draw water with it: **more urine** is then passed.

e) Passing more urine draws on the body's fluid reserves, and causes **thirst** in an attempt by the body to replace the lost fluid.

f) Excessive urination also results in loss of essential chemicals, producing **cramps, tiredness, weakness, and weight loss**.

g) If severe loss of fluid occurs in the urine, the body becomes dry (**dehydration**): breathlessness and even coma may then occur. Fortunately this is uncommon in your type of diabetes.

# 5 WHAT IS A NORMAL BLOOD GLUCOSE LEVEL?

In people without diabetes, the fasting blood glucose level (after not eating overnight) is less than 5 millimoles per litre, or 90 milligrams per decilitre (shortened to mmol/l or mg/dl). After food, it rarely rises above 8 mmol/l (145 mg/dl). In untreated or uncontrolled diabetes it can rise to 30 mmol/l (540 mg/dl) or even higher. Your doctor will probably aim to keep your blood glucose level less than 10 mmol/l (180 mg/dl) for most of the time and in some cases will help you to

Normal variation of blood glucose in a non-diabetic person.

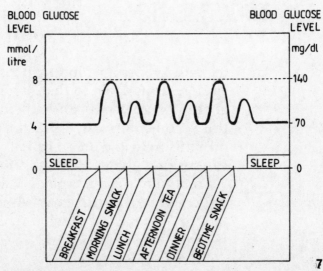

achieve the lower (more normal) levels mentioned above. It is important to realise that the symptoms of diabetes (see Question 4) are unlikely to occur unless your blood glucose is consistently higher than 14 mmol/l (250 mg/dl).

Therefore, **just because you feel well, it does not necessarily indicate that your diabetes is controlled.**

## 6 DOES DIABETES EVER GO AWAY?

No. It can always be controlled and with treatment you should feel completely well. Even when treated, however, it must still be carefully watched by you and regularly reviewed by your doctor for the rest of your life.

## 7 WHAT ARE THE MAJOR AIMS AND PRINCIPLES OF DIABETIC TREATMENT?

The first aim of treating your diabetes is to keep your blood glucose level as close as possible to that of a non-diabetic person. By this and other means, the second aim can be achieved: to minimise or avoid the so-called complications of diabetes (see Question 22).

Treatment of your type of diabetes is quite simple - particularly when overweight is a factor. Such increase in weight is due mainly to a combination of eating more food than the body needs, together with insufficient exercise, although some people certainly do seem to gain weight more easily than others. You have an excellent chance of treating your diabetes by eating less (and perhaps better quality) food, (see Questions 8 and 9) and by exercising more (see Question 11). Your doctor will arrange for you to see a dietitian for advice on the food you should include in your daily diet.

Sometimes it is necessary to prescribe additional tablets to achieve full control of your diabetes. This will be discussed later (see Question 13).

## 8/ WHAT IS A DIABETIC DIET?

A diabetic diet is a healthy, balanced diet. It is the sort of diet that is recommended for everyone (except children under five). Why not convert your family and friends?

A dietitian will probably advise you on a diet suitable for you. However, there are some basic principles which all people with diabetes should follow, both to lose weight (if necessary) and to keep their diabetes well controlled. There are six main principles:

a) **Avoid sugar and sugary foods**
We are talking about sugar, glucose, jam, honey, sweets, chocolates, fizzy drinks, and fruit squashes. The sugar

in these foods enters the blood very quickly, causing a rapid rise in blood sugar. Many foods contain sugar. However, it is only necessary to avoid foods in which sugar is a major ingredient. Check the ingredient label of a food if you are not sure it is suitable. The ingredients are listed in order of weight: i.e. sugar at the top of the list means it contains a large amount. If sugar is towards the end of the list, then the food is suitable: i.e. it contains very little.

b) **Eat regularly**
You should aim for three meals a day, rather than one or two large ones. A meal may be as little as a sandwich, or as much as a cooked meal of meat, potatoes and vegetables, followed by dessert. Eating regularly is particularly important if you have to take medication (i.e. tablets) for your diabetes, as your blood sugar may go too low if you miss a meal.

c) **Eat some starchy food with each meal**
We are talking about bread, potatoes, rice, pasta, and breakfast cereal. In earlier years, diabetics were advised to avoid or restrict these foods. We now believe that a good intake of them is important. These foods are broken down into sugar by the body. They are broken down more slowly than sugary foods, causing a slower, smaller rise in blood sugar. These sorts of changes in blood sugar also occur in non-diabetic people and are thus, to some extent,

normal. Eat the amount of starchy foods you normally have with a meal: ie. two slices of bread, two potatoes, etc.

### d)  Eat less fat and fatty foods

We are including here butter, oil, margarine, fried foods, and pastry of all types. People with diabetes are rather more likely than the average to have heart disease or strokes. Having a high fat intake increases your risk of developing these problems. Other risk factors include smoking, being overweight, and having high blood pressure. It makes sense to avoid risks! Cutting down on fat has the added advantage that it automatically reduces your calorie intake, as high fat foods are more fattening than lower fat alternatives. Avoiding high fat foods will therefore help you to reduce your weight, if necessary, or help to prevent you from becoming overweight.

### e)  Drink alcohol in moderation

The safe weekly limits are considered to be 15 drinks (or units) for a woman, or 22 drinks (or units) for a man, spread over the week. One unit is a single pub measure of spirit, an average glass of wine, or a half pint of beer, lager or cider. Alcohol is high in calories and will make you gain weight. It is also bad for your general health (liver, heart, brain, and nerves, in particular) if taken in excess. Too much alcohol at once, especially on an empty stomach, may cause your blood sugar to go too low ("hypo"). Do *not* drink on an empty stomach, avoid having more than three or four drinks in a session, and follow alcohol with a snack containing starchy food, such as a sandwich.

f) **Eat more fibre**

Dietary fibre is the part of a plant which is not digested properly by the body. High fibre foods include wholemeal bread, brown rice, wholegrain pasta, vegetables (especially beans, peas, and lentils) and wholegrain breakfast cereals. Eating high fibre foods with your meals reduces the rise in blood sugar which occurs after eating. High fibre foods can also be helpful in reducing blood fats, i.e. cholesterol, and tend to be very filling. They can therefore be helpful in reducing weight and preventing weight gain. They also help to produce regular bowel movements. Keeping your weight down has been mentioned many times in this Section. Turn to Question 10 to see the desirable weight for you. It is *very* important that you try to reduce your weight if you are overweight.

Diabetes is more difficult to control when you are overweight. If you are having difficulty in losing weight, ask your doctor to refer you to a dietitian. He or she will draw up an eating plan tailored to your needs which will help you to achieve your weight target. As we learn more about diabetes, some changes to your diet my prove necessary. It is important that you keep in touch with your dietitian, who will be able to keep you up to date. See Question 30 and check that you have the correct contact number.

## 9 / WHAT FOODS CAN I EAT?

**Foods to have freely:**

*Vegetables:* All vegetables (including baked beans) except for olives and avocado pears, which are high in fat. Vegetables are high in fibre, relatively low in calories, and a good source of vitamins and minerals. They are also one of the few things that you can eat more of if you need to lose weight!

*Fruits:* Blackberries, blackcurrants, loganberries, gooseberries, red-currants, grapefruit, lemon, melon (all varieties), and rhubarb. All other fruits should be taken in moderation, i.e. *one at a time.* You could have an apple, an orange, and a banana a day, if you wish; just remember not to have them all at once. Pure fruit juice, regardless of whether it is sweetened or not will cause your blood sugar to rise quickly. Restrict it to a quarter of a pint (150ml), at the most, at a time.

*Drinks:* Tea, coffee, diet or low calorie drinks, tomato juice, soda water, mineral waters (and tap water), thin soups, Bovril and Oxo.

*Seasonings:* Herbs, spices, salt (in moderation), vinegar, tomato puree, stock cubes, etc.

*Sweetening agents:* Artificial sweeteners, e.g. saccharin, Canderel, Sweetex, etc. Sweetening agents made by using a combination of sugar and sweetener, e.g. Sucron, should be avoided.

**Foods to have in your usual amounts:**
*Starchy foods:* Remember to have them at each meal. Recommended high fibre breakfast cereals are - porridge, branflakes, Weetabix, shredded wheat, etc. Cereals with "no added sugar" written on the label will be suitable. Other starchy foods include potatoes, yam, cassava, plantain, sweet potato, rice, pasta, bread, crackers, nans, pittas, chapattis – especially the wholemeal or wholegrain varieties.

**Foods to have in moderation:**
*Fat:* The following fats are very fatty and therefore should only be taken in small amounts – lard, butter, oil (including polyunsaturated and olive oil), margarine. Other foods can also make your fat intake higher than it should be, e.g. hidden fats in pastry, batter, salad dressings. There is also hidden fat in cheese, meat, eggs, poultry and fish. These foods should therefore be taken in small portions and cooked without adding further fat, i.e. grilled, poached, steamed or baked.

# IS WEIGHT CONTROL IMPORTANT?

Yes. Being over-weight increases your body's need for insulin and can make your diabetes less stable. It may also cause or aggravate conditions unrelated to diabetes, such as high blood pressure and arthritis.

The only way you can influence your weight is by diet and exercise (see Question 11). Remember that one extra hour of brisk walking (or half- an-hour of continuous swimming, jogging or

## ADULT DESIRABLE WEIGHT
A weight 2–2.5 kg (5 pounds) above or below is acceptable!

| HEIGHT (without shoes) | | WEIGHT (without clothes) | | | |
| | | MEN | | WOMEN | |
| Feet/ Inches | Centi- metres | Pounds | Kilo- grams | Pounds | Kilo- grams |
| --- | --- | --- | --- | --- | --- |
| 4/10 | 147.5 | — | — | 107 | 48.5 |
| 4/11 | 150.0 | — | — | 110 | 50.0 |
| 5/0 | 152.5 | — | — | 113 | 51.5 |
| 5/1 | 155.0 | — | — | 116 | 52.5 |
| 5/2 | 157.5 | 129 | 58.5 | 119 | 54.0 |
| 5/3 | 160.0 | 133 | 60.5 | 122 | 55.5 |
| 5/4 | 162.5 | 136 | 62.0 | 126 | 57.0 |
| 5/5 | 165.0 | 139 | 63.0 | 130 | 59.0 |
| 5/6 | 167.5 | 143 | 65.0 | 135 | 61.0 |
| 5/7 | 170.0 | 147 | 66.5 | 139 | 63.0 |
| 5/8 | 172.5 | 152 | 69.0 | 143 | 65.0 |
| 5/9 | 175.5 | 156 | 71.0 | 147 | 66.5 |
| 5/10 | 178.0 | 160 | 72.5 | 151 | 68.5 |
| 5/11 | 180.5 | 165 | 75.0 | 155 | 70.5 |
| 6/0 | 183.0 | 170 | 77.0 | — | — |
| 6/1 | 185.5 | 175 | 79.5 | — | — |
| 6/2 | 188.0 | 180 | 81.5 | — | — |
| 6/3 | 190.5 | 185 | 83.5 | — | — |
| 6/4 | 193.0 | 190 | 86.0 | — | — |

squash) each day will almost predictably allow you to lose about 7 kg (15 pounds) in a year – providing you do not increase your food intake! Use the table on p.15 as a guide to your goal weight.

A weight 2-2.5 kg (5 pounds) above or below the "desirable" is acceptable!

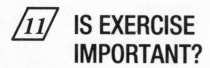

## IS EXERCISE IMPORTANT?

Yes. Any form of exercise causes the muscles to use more glucose. Not only is the blood glucose level lowered immediately after exercise, but there appears to be a long term lowering of blood glucose levels in people whose lifestyle is more energetic. Most people do not realise how inactive they really are. Tiredness and fatigue after a day's work are due more to emotional stress and tension than to the effects of muscular exercise.

Any type of exercise is satisfactory for diabetics, including cycling, regular sport, or just plain walking. A careful look at your lifestyle and discussion with friends and family should help you plan a more energetic way of life, whatever your age or other medical problems.

## WHAT IF DIET AND EXERCISE ALONE ARE NOT SUFFICIENT?

Provided that your symptoms are not severe, your doctor and dietitian will probably persevere for days or even weeks just watching the effects of their advice on diet and exercise, particularly if you are much overweight. If control is not achieved in this way (as shown by consistently high urine or blood glucose levels), or if your first symptoms are quite severe, additional tablets will be prescribed. Unfortunately, insulin itself cannot be taken by mouth, since it is destroyed by enzymes in the stomach and bowel.

## 13/ HOW DO "ANTI-DIABETIC" TABLETS (ORAL HYPOGLYCAEMIC DRUGS) ACT?

There are three main groups, the most common of which are called sulphonylurea drugs. The names of those most frequently used are as follows (proprietary names in brackets):

| | |
|---|---|
| tolbutamide | (Rastinon, Pramidex, Artosin) |
| chlorpropamide | (Diabenese) |
| glibenclamide | (Euglucon, Daonil) |
| gliquidone | (Glurenorm) |
| acetohexamide | (Dimelor) |
| glipizide | (Glibenese, Minodiab) |
| tolazamide | (Tolanase) |
| gliclazide | (Diamicron) |

All of these drugs act partly by stimulating the pancreas to produce more insulin, and partly by improving the action of whatever insulin is already being produced. It is now considered that some of these drugs may have other effects which benefit diabetes. These are still under study.

The second group of drugs are called biguanides, the only one currently in use being metformin (Glucophage). This acts by improving the action of any insulin you are still producing, directly helping glucose to enter tissue cells.

The third group of drugs are called alpha-glucosidase inhibitors, the current main member of which is called acarbose (Glucobay). These drugs act by slowing down the breakdown of complex carbohydrates like starches, so that the glucose which results from the breakdown will be absorbed more slowly.

## 14/ CAN TABLETS EVER PRODUCE SIDE EFFECTS?

Yes. All sulphonylureas when given in too high a dose can cause the blood glucose level to drop too far (hypoglycaemia, or "hypo"). This may produce a feeling of hunger, dizziness, slurred speech, trembling, sweating, faintness, or even loss of consciousness. The blood glucose level usually drops to below 2.5 mmol/l (45 mg/dl) in someone who is having a hypo.

Clearly, if you miss a meal, a "hypo" is more likely to occur and irregular or missed meals must particularly be avoided with glibenclamide and chlorpropamide.

All drugs very occasionally produce a rash, and in many people taking chlor-propamide, even a small alcoholic drink can produce a hot flush. If this occurs, tell your doctor, and he can change you to a different tablet in the same group - or you may prefer to keep off alcoholic drinks!

Metformin hardly ever lowers the blood glucose too far, unless used in combination with a sulphonylurea drug, but it can produce a feeling of sickness, stomach discomfort, or diar-rhoea. If this happens, contact your doctor. Very rarely it can produce seri-ous illness, particularly if you have other heart, liver, kidney, or blood ves-sel problems. Your doctor will regularly check for these other problems and will not prescribe metformin if any are present.

Acarbose (Glucobay) may produce excessive wind. Other than this it is quite safe.

# WHAT HAPPENS IF THE TABLETS DO NOT WORK?

You must first ask yourself if you are still keeping to the diet-and-exercise programme prescribed for you. Remember that the tablets are not substitutes for this programme.

If you are doing all the right things and control is still poor, your doctor may suggest an increased tablet dose or a change of tablets, perhaps adding metformin or acarbose to a sulphonylurea drug, or he may recommend insulin injections.

Commencing on insulin is not a calamity. Often you will actually feel very much better once insulin is begun. Sometimes your doctor may add a dose of insulin to your tablets either in the morning or in the evening. Sometimes insulin is given instead of the tablets. The routine of giving injections every day can be rapidly mastered even by the most elderly patient, perhaps with the help of a district nurse or relative. Ask your doctor for the companion volume to this book, which deals with insulin-dependent-diabetes, if insulin is in fact needed.

## 16/ HOW CAN ONE TELL WHETHER DIABETES IS ACTUALLY CONTROLLED?

By the way you feel? No! This can be most unreliable. Many diabetics may feel perfectly well despite uncontrolled diabetes: yet this can produce undesirable effects over time (see Question 22). The symptoms listed in Question 4 should be well recognised by you: if they occur, your diabetes is badly out of control! The cause must be found and corrected immediately.

**By testing the urine?** Yes! All diabetics should at least test their own urine, ideally once or more each day. Positive tests usually mean that the diabetes has not been well controlled during the previous four or five hours. Even negative tests may not give the whole picture: blood glucose can be high without it showing up in the urine (see Question 18).

**By testing the blood?** Yes! Measuring the blood glucose levels is the most direct way of checking how good the control of your diabetes really is. You can do these tests yourself, as explained later, again ideally once or twice each day.

The diagram on page 7 gave you an idea how blood glucose levels rise in response to food, and return to normal as the body's insulin takes effect in a person who does not have diabetes.

In a person with diabetes, a blood glucose level which is below 10 mmol/l (180 mg/dl) is a good target. Your doctor may however advise you to aim for blood glucose levels rather lower than this: you should always be aware what your personal targets are, by discussing the matter with your doctor.

**By testing the haemoglobin A1?** This is a blood test which is taken by your doctor or nurse and analysed by the laboratory. The result of the test gives an estimate of how well your diabetes has been controlled over the previous month or two. Ask your doctor what your level is, so that you know how you are getting on with your control. Levels above 8% usually mean that there is room for improvement!

## 17 HOW DOES ONE TEST THE URINE?

**Clinistix (or Testape):** These dip-strips only tell you whether or not glucose is present in the urine. They are quite inaccurate for finding out the actual amount and are therefore unsatisfactory for routine use by diabetics.

**Diabur-5000 or Diastix** dip-strips show a clearer and more definite colour change, depending on exactly how much glucose is present in the urine. They are quite satisfactory for routine use. The result should be recorded as 0, 1/10th, 1%, etc.

Whichever test is used, it is most important that you follow the instructions very carefully: although they are simple to do, you can still get a wrong answer if you don't do the test carefully! A number of drugs taken in high dosage, including vitamin C and aspirin, interfere with the colour reaction of all these tests. They can make the tests look lower than they actually are. Check with your doctor that the medication which you take regularly is not likely to interfere with the tests in this way.

# 18 WHAT DOES GLUCOSE IN THE URINE REALLY MEAN?

Consider the glucose levels in blood to be like water in a tank.

When it reaches a certain level (the threshold), it overflows into the urine. In most people this threshold is above 8 mmol/l (140 mg/dl) (A in the figure above). This is the highest blood glucose level reached by most non-diabetics (and well controlled diabetics). **Therefore, absence of glucose in the urine usually means good diabetic control: the worse the control, the more glucose will appear in the urine.**

However, your threshold may be low (B in figure): then the sugar may be present in the urine even with a normal blood glucose level.

Finally, your threshold may be high (C in the figure). Then the blood glucose levels can be quite high without it

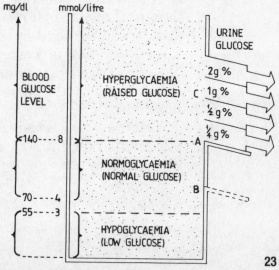

showing up in the urine: you will therefore be misled into thinking that your diabetes is well controlled. It is partly for these reasons that your doctor may advise you to test your blood rather than your urine. It is also worth remembering that people without diabetes do not have sugar in their urine: ideally, you should be aiming for this target too!

## 19 HOW DOES ONE TEST THE BLOOD?

Quite a simple and almost painless method of pricking your finger yourself now exists and can be shown to you by your doctor or nurse. A drop of blood put on the end of a special glucose testing strip (e.g. BM 1-44 or Glucostix) allows quite an accurate assessment of your blood glucose level. You can quite easily do this yourself, although you must be careful to get a good drop of blood (not a smear). It is also essential that you wipe the blood off the strip at exactly the right time recommended by the manufacturers, otherwise an inaccurate result is obtained. Meters are available to give a number (digital) read-out of your sugar level.

Whichever test is used, it is most important that you follow the instructions very carefully.

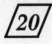 # WHEN SHOULD URINE OR BLOOD BE TESTED?

Preferably every day. First thing in the morning (or before a meal) is the time when glucose in blood and urine is likely to be at its lowest level: one to two hours after the main meal of the day is the time when the glucose level is likely to be at its highest. Both these measurements are important, and your doctor will recommend one or more tests spread throughout the day, to get a clear picture of what is going on. It is essential that you write the test results down in a record book and bring this either to the clinic or to your doctor's surgery each time you visit. By doing this, the doctor or nurse can see how well you are controlled and can provide suggestions as to how control may be improved.

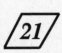 # WHAT CAN CAUSE DIABETES TO GO OUT OF CONTROL?

There are many things which affect the blood glucose level: the tug of war diagram on the next page will help remind you of the most important ones. If you keep this "tug-of-war" in mind, it will help to keep your diabetes under control.

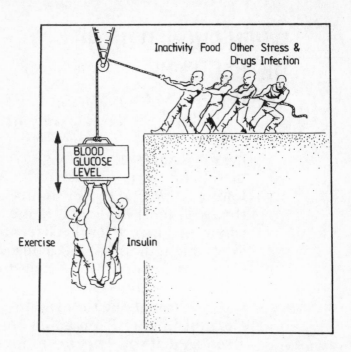

It is most important to remember that even a slight infection like a bad cold or an emotional upset can affect your control quite badly, and this will show up as a positive urine test or a high blood sugar level. Emotional stresses do the same thing. If your tests are still high after a couple of days, contact your doctor or Hotline number: you may need a bigger dose of tablets or even a short course of insulin until the problem settles down.

**WHAT ARE THE SO-CALLED COMPLICATIONS OF DIABETES?**

**Arteriosclerosis** (hardening of the arteries) occurs to some extent in almost every person as they age, whether they are diabetic or not. In some diabetics, it may occur somewhat earlier than usual. Arteriosclerosis is the cause of stroke and heart attacks. It may also produce poor circulation in the legs which leads to painful calves on walking, ulcers on the feet, and occasionally gangrene.

Hardening of the arteries is caused by fat being deposited in the walls of the arteries, so that they become narrowed, and even blocked. From time to time, your doctor will check the level of cholesterol (as well as other fats) in your blood. Keeping these blood fat levels normal reduces the risk of developing heart attacks and strokes. The way to keep the fat levels normal is to keep to the recommended diet (see Questions 8 & 9). Somewhat stricter dieting and even medicines may be prescribed for you if the fats in the blood test are found to be above safe levels.

*Diabetics should not smoke:* smoking is the other big cause of hardening of the arteries.

If arteries do become blocked, they

can quite often be treated by a surgeon stretching or bypassing the block. But, prevention is better than cure!

**Cataracts** are degenerative changes in the lens of the eye which can cause dimness of vision. Cataracts occur commonly in non-diabetics and somewhat more frequently in diabetics, especially if blood sugar levels are allowed to run high. Cataract can be treated by quite a simple operation: the faulty lens is removed, and an artificial one inserted by the surgeon at the time of the operation.

**Retinopathy** is the name given to leaky and abnormally fragile small blood vessels in the retina, the seeing part of the eye. Such abnormalities may cause blurring, and occasionally actual loss of vision.

It is your responsibility to make sure that a doctor (or suitably qualified optician) checks the retina of the eye every year with an ophthalmoscope. Even once retinopathy has developed, it can usually be effectively treated by using laser beam therapy ... unless it is left too late!

**Neuropathy** signifies nerve damage, which can cause weakness, pins and needles, or a loss of feeling in the hands or feet, and occasionally dizziness and other unusual symptoms. It is important to realise that you may not know that you have a loss of feeling in the feet: only a regular check by your doctor will make it possible to pick this problem up in its earliest form. Even a lack of sexual performance can occur, although this may be due to factors other than diabetes.

**Nephropathy** means kidney damage, which may occur after long-standing diabetes. It is for this reason that your doctor checks for protein in your urine when you visit him: if present, it may be an early sign of this problem.

**High blood pressure** occurs rather more often in people with diabetes. It can increase the risk of heart attacks and strokes, and can also worsen retinopathy and nephropathy. You must make sure that your doctor or nurse checks your blood pressure at least once a year. Quite simple tablet treatment is now available for this problem. If you are already taking blood pressure tablets, it is important that you have your pressure checked at least every 3 months. It is quite important for you to know what your blood pressure is, and what your doctor would like it to be. In general, a blood pressure of above 160/90 is not considered to be healthy in the long term.

**Infection**, particularly of the skin and urinary system, is more likely to occur in diabetics than in people without diabetes. In addition, healing of even minor injuries is sometimes slower.

All these complications can be effectively treated, particularly if detected early. It is for this reason that the doctor will make a systematic examination of various parts of your body approximately once each year. You may need to remind him that this annual review is due! Keeping your diabetes well controlled is also one way that you yourself can help reduce the risk of these complications.

**Foot Ulcers** are a particular risk. If feeling is lost, it is all too easy to be unaware of pressure on a toe or a minor injury. Repeated damage to this area, particularly if your blood circulation is poor can then result in an ulcer. This can become more infected, producing swelling, redness and pain, and loss of control of your diabetes. You could become seriously ill, and even gangrene may develop, requiring amputation of part of your foot. Chronic ulcer infection can also damage the underlying bone (osteomyelitis). Once this sets in, long-term antibiotic treatment or surgery to your foot may prove necessary. Prevention is all important: please read the answer to Question 24 very carefully. If you develop even the smallest ulcer or sore on the foot, let your doctor know immediately.

## 23 DOES EVERY DIABETIC GET COMPLICATIONS AT SOME TIME?

No. There is good evidence that most of the above complications are less likely to occur if the diabetes is well controlled, and if weight gain is avoided. However, it must be admitted that even the best controlled diabetic does sometimes have one or other of the complications mentioned above.

 **HOW IMPORTANT IS FOOT CARE?** A diabetic's feet can be very vulnerable.

Nerve damage (neuropathy) can prevent feeling an injury, scratch, or cut; poor blood supply to the feet may then mean poor healing of the injury and infection or gangrene can develop, as mentioned above.

The following rules are important to follow:

a) Avoid walking bare-foot, even at home.

b) Do not cut your toenails too short, and cut nails to follow the line of the toe.

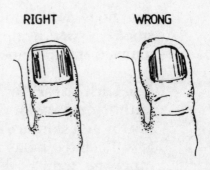

RIGHT          WRONG

c) Never cut your own toenails if you have a significant eye-sight problem, or a nerve or blood vessel disorder affecting the feet: see a state registered chiropodist regularly every 6-8 weeks, if possible.

d) Avoid tight shoes: preferably have new shoes fitted by an expert who knows you are diabetic.

e) Wash, dry, and examine your feet carefully at least every other day: even the most minor infection should be immediately discussed with your doctor.

f) Never attempt to treat any foot problem yourself. Permanent damage may result from the use of "over the counter" remedies: always seek professional advice first.

## 25/ A FEW ADDITIONAL QUESTIONS

**Can I smoke?** Diabetes alone may damage the blood vessels of your body, as mentioned earlier. If you smoke as well, your chances of such damage are that much greater.

**Can I drive a car?** Yes, but the licensing authorities may want to have your doctor's reassurance that your diabetes is sufficiently stable, and that you are otherwise well: an appropriate form will need to be completed, on which you must mention that you have diabetes.

**Can I play sport?** Yes. See Questions 10 and 11.

**Can I drink alcohol?** Yes, but as mentioned earlier, weight control is very important and alcoholic drinks add to your calorie intake. In addition, if you are prone to having "hypos", alcohol (especially spirits) may block the body's corrective responses, and make your "hypos" more severe. Remember that you should always have a starchy snack if you have an alcoholic drink.

**Does diabetes interfere with employment?** Hardly. Jobs involving physical responsibility for other people (e.g. bus drivers, airline pilots, certain branches of the armed forces), may be a problem if you are taking the sulphonylurea group of drugs or insulin (which are the only drugs which can produce hypos). Apart from these situations, there should be no problems. The earlier discrimination against diabetics is now almost non-existent since it has been shown that the work record of diabetics is on average better than that of non-diabetics.

**Can I get life insurance?** Yes. You may have to accept a "loading", but life insurance is possible for most diabetics. Shop around and seek the advice of your Diabetic Association office.

**What about children?** If you are a woman in the child-bearing age group, you will be advised to be absolutely sure that your diabetes is perfectly controlled before becoming pregnant: wait until your doctor gives you the go-ahead. Once you are pregnant, you will probably need to have insulin injections for much of the pregnancy in order to achieve the level of control known to be important to get a healthy baby. Insulin can be discontinued again in most people after the confinement. Diabetes is at least partly inherited. If either parent is a diabetic, the risk of any one child becoming diabetic at some time of their life is certainly greater. In your type of diabetes it is worth suggesting to your children that they be regularly checked for diabetes once they are above 40 years of age. It is also sensible for them to strenuously avoid becoming overweight, which could trigger off their diabetes.

**Pregnancy** in a diabetic should always be managed by a physician/obstetrician team accustomed to dealing with diabetic pregnancies: a lot of emphasis will be placed on making sure that your diabetes is well controlled.

**Contraception**: Most of the presently available low-dose pills are satisfactory for diabetics and there is no reason why you cannot use intra-uterine devices (IUD) or other contraceptive methods. If you are "on the pill", it is useful to stop it and to have one normal period before you conceive, so that the exact stage of pregnancy is known. Your physicians will be happy to discuss other aspects of diabetes and pregnancy with you.

## 27 WHEN SHOULD I SEE MY DOCTOR OR CLINIC?

**Routinely:** Ideally you should have a discussion with a doctor or nurse at least every 4 months. Do not forget to take your test record book with you when you go.

At about yearly intervals and perhaps more frequently, your doctor will systematically examine your eyes, blood pressure, heart, blood vessels of the feet, and check for nerve damage. He will not mind if you remind him that your 12 months check is due. He or she will test the urine for protein, and check the level of control of your diabetes and your kidney function. A blood sample may also be taken to see whether the blood fat (cholesterol and triglyceride) levels are normal. An alteration to the diet, and perhaps tablets, may be suggested if they are not.

As indicated earlier, a number of drugs in everyday use for other conditions may affect the control of your diabetes, or interfere with the strip tests. Therefore, at these visits ask your doctor for reassurance that any of the other drugs that you are taking are not interfering in some way.

**In an emergency:** If your tests show high sugar levels consistently, or if you

35

begin to feel thirsty or unwell, do not wait: get advice. Make sure that you have one or more telephone numbers that you or your family or friends may contact for advice on such unexpected problems, and write them down in the space provided on page 37 (Question 30 "Hotline") for easy reference. Your doctor may have given you another type of test strip (Ketostix) to measure ketones in the urine. Ketones will appear in the urine when fat is broken down to provide reserve energy. This may happen even in a non-diabetic who has not eaten for twelve hours or so. More important though, ketones appear in the urine of diabetics when control becomes really poor. Therefore, if you have consistently high glucose levels in urine or blood tests, it is a good idea to test for ketones. If positive, you would be well advised to contact your doctor or hotline immediately.

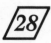 **IDENTIFICATION** Always carry a card, or better still, a bracelet or pendant, indicating that you are a diabetic. In this day and age, accidents will happen, and it is obviously important that anyone can immediately identify you as being diabetic.

The Medicalert Foundation (local address available from your doctor), which provides identification bracelets and pendants at a modest cost, now has branches in many countries. This system is highly recommended. Alternatively, have your local jeweller make up one for you.

## 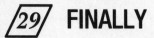 FINALLY

Remember that knowing about your diabetes is your responsibility. Your physician, dietitian, clinic sister, or chiropodist/podiatrist will be only too happy to answer queries and suggest further reading material.

Membership of the British Diabetic Association has much to offer. It can help you follow recent trends in diabetes care. Much research is also being carried out into diabetes, including new methods of treating the problem. You will find it useful and interesting to keep in touch with these important developments.

## /30/ "HOTLINE"

In this space you should write down a telephone number, from which you can get advice 24 hours a day, seven days a week, should any sudden problem occur which affects your diabetes. Your doctor or nurse will advise you which number to insert.

..............................................................

## /31/ OTHER IMPORTANT CONTACT NUMBERS

Your family doctor.........................................................

Your clinic appointment clerk.....................................

Your dietitian ...............................................................

Your chiropodist/podiatrist........................................

Your diabetic advisory service ...................................

 **SOME BOOKS FOR FURTHER READING:**

*Non-insulin Dependent Handbook,* by John Day, Suzanne Redmond and Sue Brenchley. Publishers: Medikos.

*Diabetes at your Fingertips,* by Peter Sonksen, Charles Fox and Sue Judd. Publishers: Class Publishing.

*Diabetes- a Basic Guide,* by Rowan Hillson. Publishers: McDonald Optima

# INDEX